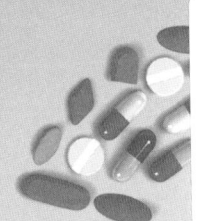

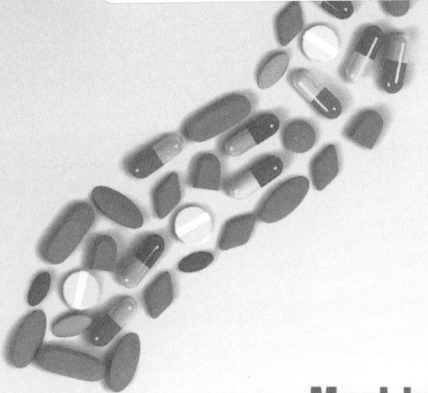

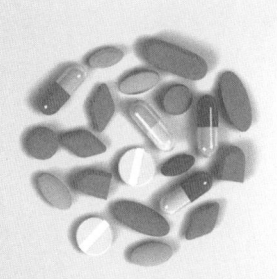

Must-know Health Facts

R. J. B. Willis

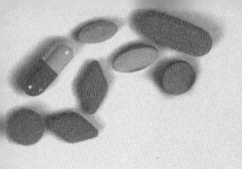

First published in 2010

Copyright © 2010 Autumn House (Europe) Ltd

All rights reserved. No part of this publication may be reproduced in any form without prior permission from the publishers.

British Library Cataloguing in Publication Data. A catalogue record for this book is available from the British Library.

ISBN 978-1-906381-76-9

Published by Autumn House (Europe) Ltd, Grantham, Lincolnshire.

Designed by Abigail Murphy.

Printed in Thailand.

Bible versions used, indicated by initials:

NIV = *New International Version* (Hodder and Stoughton)

NCV = *New Century Version* (Thomas Nelson)

Circular chuckles

'I don't laugh because I'm happy,
I'm happy because I laugh.'
Dr Carl Simonton

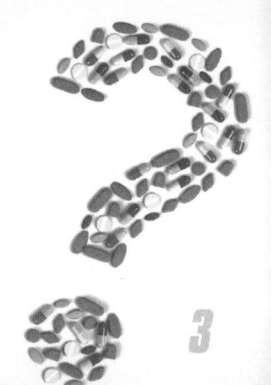

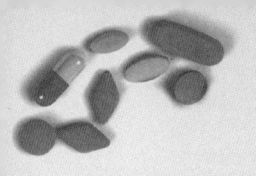

Laugh yourself well

'A cheerful heart is good medicine.'
Proverbs 17:22, NIV

An inexpensive cure

'Always laugh when you can.
It is cheap medicine.'

Lord Byron

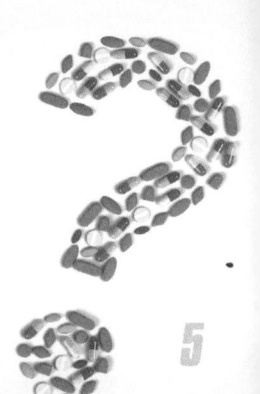

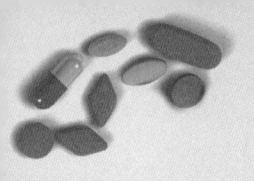

Time to smile

'... laughter may serve as a blocking agent, a sort of bullet-proof vest that can help protect an individual against the ravages of negative emotions that arise with disease.'

Dr William F. Fry

The hostile womb

The more painkillers a woman takes during labour, the greater the likelihood of the child abusing drugs later on in life. A child is nearly five times more likely to abuse drugs if the mother received *opiates* or *barbiturates* in the hours before birth.

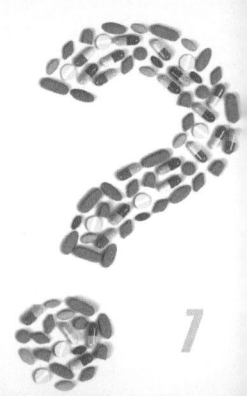

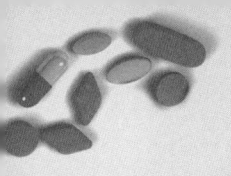

The cost of booze

Alcohol-related crime and insurance figures are in excess of £142 million in the UK.

Alcohol is a factor in:
- ⅓ of domestic accidents
- ⅕ of all drownings
- ⅔ of suicides
- ½ of all murders
- 80% of fire deaths
- ⅓ of child abuse cases

High cal alcohol

A poll of 2,000 UK adults showed that four in ten did not know the calorific value of their alcoholic drink:
- a glass of red wine = a slice of sponge cake
- a pint of beer/lager = a small sausage roll
- a pint of cider = a portion of beans on toast
- a cream liqueur = a chicken drumstick
- spirit drinks = a 25ml serving of single cream

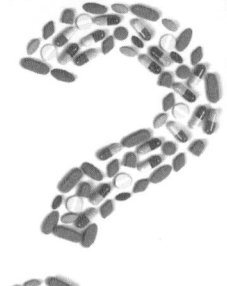

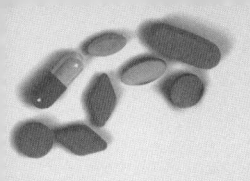

The grapes of wrath?

'A hangover is the wrath of grapes.'
Author unknown

'Wine and beer make people loud and uncontrolled; it is not wise to get drunk on them.'
Proverbs 20:1, NCV

The folly of drink

'When the wine is in, the wit is out.'
Proverb

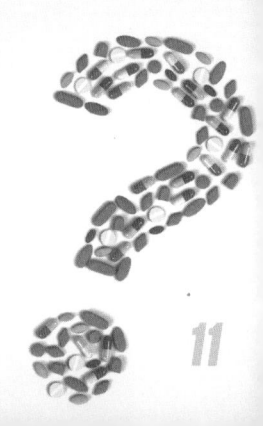

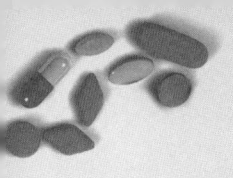

The agony of ecstasy

Five hundred thousand *ecstasy* takers worldwide are affected by:
- brain damage
- impaired intellectual ability
- changes in mood and personality
- increased risk of psychiatric conditions
- diminished appetite and dehydration

More on ecstasy

There are:
- 450,000 regular users in the US
- 500,000 who take it each year in the UK
- heavy users who take up to 40,000 tablets in a lifetime of ecstasy use

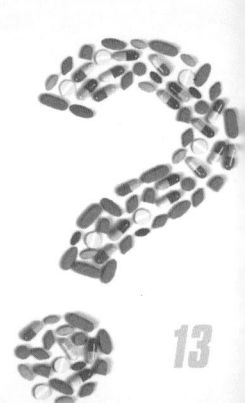

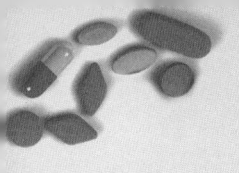

Ecstatic or incensed?

JWHO 18 – a synthetic drug which mimics the main active ingredient of *cannabis* with an effect five times more powerful – is being sold legally as part of incense and is not subject to the same legal restraints. Some countries have already banned its use.

Drug highs

- 27% of British adults have taken illegal drugs, with 44% of those still using.
- Of drug users, 18% started through peer pressure, 80% out of curiosity and 2% to copy hero figures.
- 15% of drug users take drugs daily, and 34% take drugs weekly.

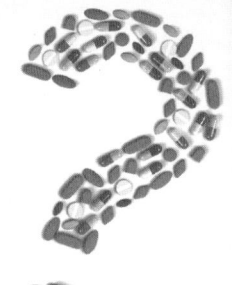

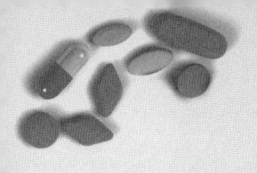

A definition of smoking

'A custom loathsome to the eye, hateful to the nose, harmful to the brain, dangerous to the lungs, and in the black, stinking fume thereof nearest resembling the horrible Stygian smoke of the pit that is bottomless.'

James I of England, A Counterblaste to Tobacco, *1604*

Fire!

'If we see you smoking we will assume you are on fire and take appropriate action.'
Douglas Adams

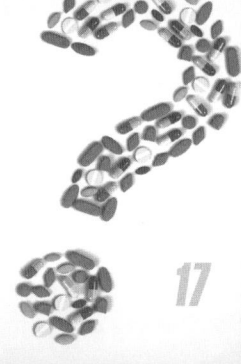

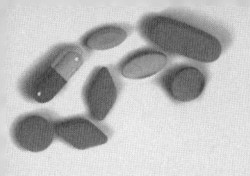

A dangerous and unwise habit

'A cigarette is a pipe with a fire at one
end and a fool at the other.'

Author unknown

A secret puff

- About 60% of pupils who currently smoke think that their parents don't know they smoke.
  - Girls are more likely to hide their smoking from their families.
  - Children are less likely to smoke if they think their parents will disapprove, even if the parents smoke.

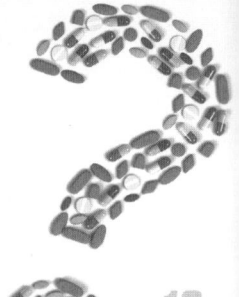

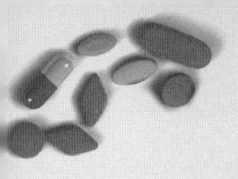

Teen smokers

- 1% of children age 11 smoke regularly, rising to 28% by age 15 for boys and 33% for girls.
  - Girls who started smoking at 16 years are regular smokers by age 19.

Passive smoking

A US government report stated: 'Maternal smoking during pregnancy and infancy is one of the most avoidable risk factors for infant death. . . . Children of parents who smoke inhale nicotine in amounts equivalent to their actively smoking 60 to 150 cigarettes per year.'

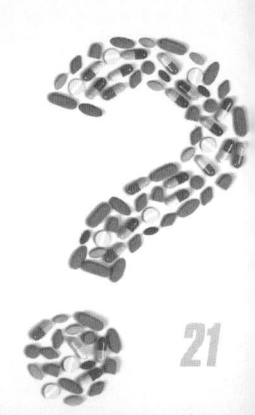

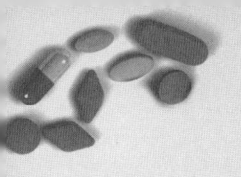

Cigarillos

Students at black universities in the US prefer cigarillos to cigarettes, believing these to be less addictive. Dr H. Jolly says: 'Tobacco prevention programmes should debunk myths that cigarillos are a safe alternative to cigarettes.'

Cadmium problems

Cadmium, a known contaminant of cigarette smoke, can increase lung disease in users of cigarettes and others exposed to passive smoking. The contaminant is also found in batteries and fertilisers and in higher levels can double the risk of *pulmonary disease*.

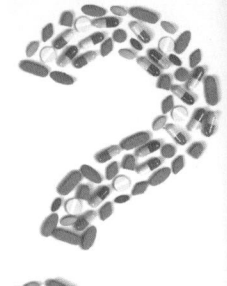

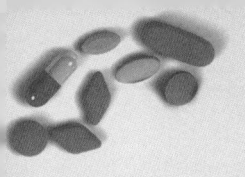

Kicking the habit

'To cease smoking is the easiest thing I ever did.
I ought to know because I've done
it a thousand times.'
Attributed to Mark Twain

Healthy ageing

'Illness is not synonymous with ageing. Many of the physical disorders that afflict seniors can be effectively treated.'
Dr Isao Horinouchi

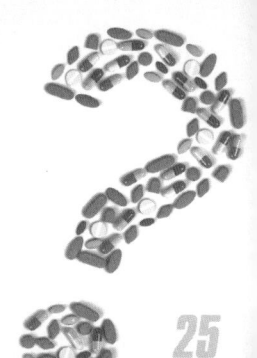

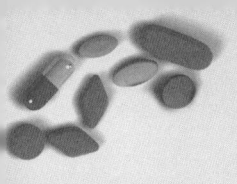

Ironing out the wrinkles

Studies from Australia, Greece and Sweden involving 450 people 70+ years of age showed that consuming a healthy diet minimised wrinkling.

The diets consisted of legumes, vegetables and low-fat milk products and were rich in *calcium, iron, magnesium, phosphorus, vitamin C* and *zinc*.

The minutia of ageing

Telomeres – the *DNA* at the end of a *chromosome* – that protect the ends from destruction and contribute to longevity, are preserved by multivitamin use.

The *telomere* length of *leukocyte* DNA was about 5.1% longer in multivitamin users, protecting the individual from *oxidative stress* and *chronic inflammation*.

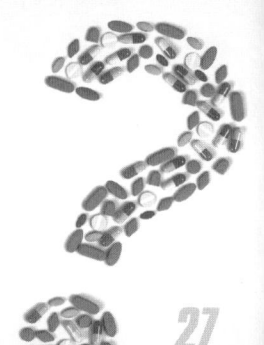

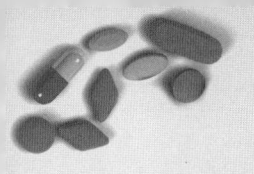

It's not all bad!

'Grow old along with me!
The best is yet to be,
The last of life, for which the first was made:
Our times are in his hand
Who saith, "A whole I planned,
Youth shows but half; trust God: see all,
nor be afraid!" '

Robert Browning

Stay young at heart!

'I want to die young at a ripe old age.'
Ashley Montagu

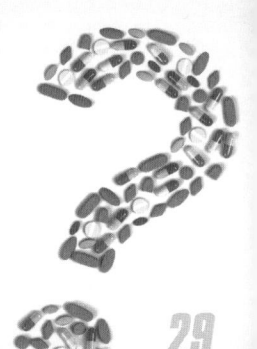

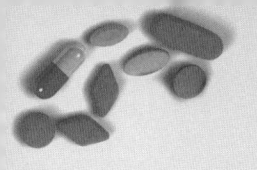

Snoring

Snoring is caused by vibration of the soft palate, the rear part of the roof of the mouth. About 10% of snoring may be due to blocked nasal passages.

Snoring kit

A wide range of anti-snoring devices is now available to the snorer:

'Some of these products may work for you, but we remain unconvinced by most of the evidence provided to support the claims.'

Emma Copeland, SNORE *researcher*

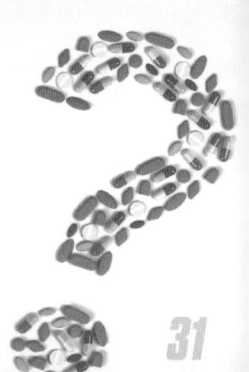

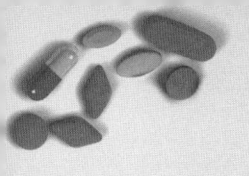

Nodding off

An American study of 3,000 women 70+ in age showed that those who sleep five or less hours a night are more likely to fall than women who sleep seven to eight hours nightly.

Benzodiazepine users were also more likely to fall.

Signs of intelligent life

People who think and act quickly have been shown to have a greater longevity chance:

'People with greater intelligence tend to have been better educated and worked in jobs where resources and workplace practices are better.'

Dr Geoff Der

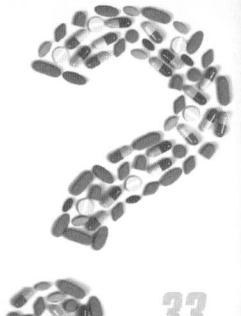

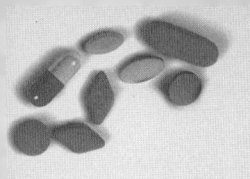

It's all downhill

It is thought that our mental powers peak at 22 and start to decline thereafter. Our reasoning, spatial visualisation and speed of thought wind down in our late 20s, although memory may stay intact until our late 30s.

Mind gym

Using a series of computerised brain training is helping *schizophrenics* with their learning, remembering and decision-making abilities, thus giving sufferers new hope for employment in the workplace. The computer programmes help the brain to make new connections.

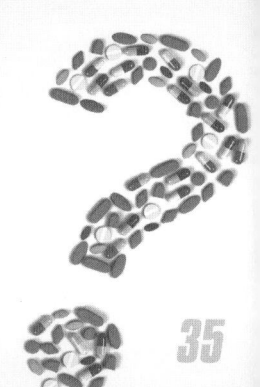

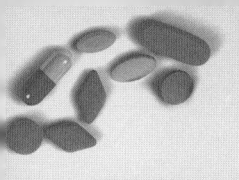

Rich brain, poor brain

Brain differences seem to separate rich and poor children. The children of higher-income families outperform their less privileged counterparts both in IQ tests and academic results. The 'rich' brain children may have higher achieving parents and other resources that aid the advantage.

Cross-wiring

Lapses in concentration or chronic boredom may be caused by parts of the brain disconnecting. Switches in focus caused new sets of connections to be made while others weakened. The normal crosstalk between regions of the brain was disrupted by the weakening and manifested itself as lapses or boredom.

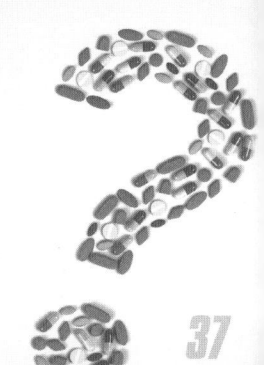

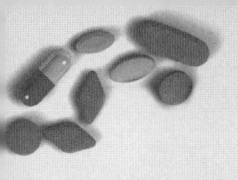

Of heart and head

Canadian scientists have discovered a region in the brain that controls the heart and blood vessels. Irregularities in the *insular cortex* give rise to hitherto unexplained heart attacks. The irregularities can be triggered by stressful incidents.

Just instinct

It would appear that subliminal messages do affect our decision-making ability. The gut reaction or instinct is quickly internalised and forms the basis of conscious decision.

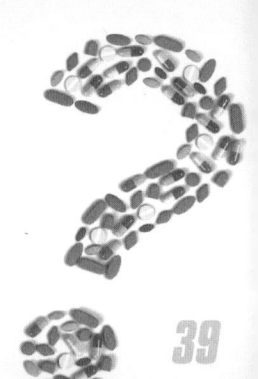

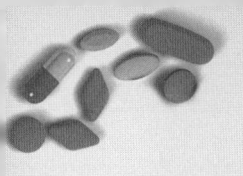

Say it with flowers

To be more specific, daffodils. A Welsh farm is growing daffodils rich in a compound *galantamine* which can slow the progress of *Alzheimer's disease*. *Galantamine* has also been extracted from snowdrops harvested in Bulgaria and China.

Cold sores

The *Journal of Pathology* reports a finding that implicates the *herpes simplex virus* (which causes cold sores) in cases of *Alzheimer's disease*.

Concentrations of the virus have been found in the *amyloid plaques* that clog the brain and are characteristic of *Alzheimer's*.

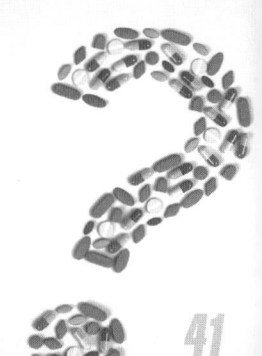

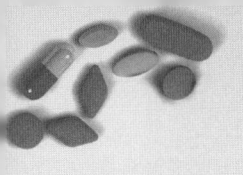

Stretching the mind

A Scottish study of 2,792 children and dating back to 1932 concluded that those with high IQs live longer. Mind-expanding games help delay the onset of *Alzheimer's* and *dementia*, thus allowing ageing with dignity.

Migraines

Migraines are felt as the arteries within the brain fill up and enlarge. The arteries of the scalp also fill up, enlarge and become rigid. The pressure caused by the enlargement on these very sensitive areas gives rise to throbbing pain and neck ache, thus adding to the discomfort.

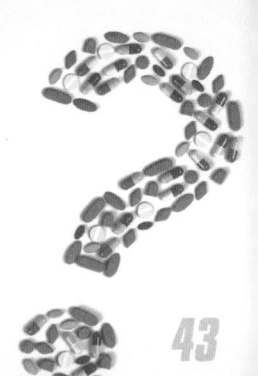

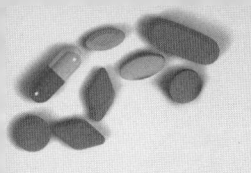

Melanoma mutation

A mutation in the *BRAF* gene can be the start of genetic changes leading to a *melanoma*. There are around 9,500 new cases of *malignant melanoma* with 2,300 deaths annually in the UK.

Nuclear families

A study in the *European Journal of Cancer Care* reported an increase in *leukaemia* rates near nuclear reactor locations.

The greatest mortality increases were in the vicinity of old reactors now closed, and about half of known cases occurred near existing plants.

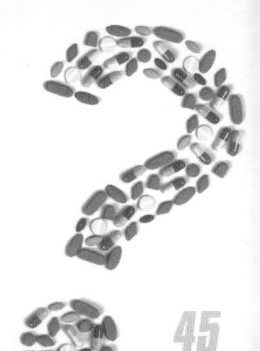

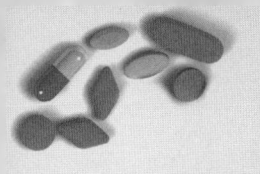

Cancer de-stress

An Ohio State University study involving 277 women recovering from *breast cancer* showed that *de-stressing* the individuals lowered the risk of relapse and extended survival.

Tea capsules

Green tea capsules promoted as anti-cancer agents may in fact contribute to the development of cancer in people taking conventional anti-cancer drugs. Drugs were inactivated by the *green tea* capsules.

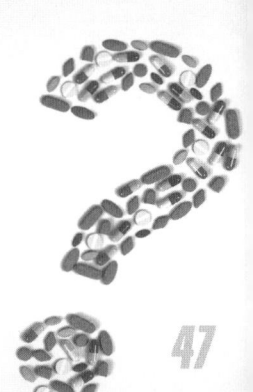

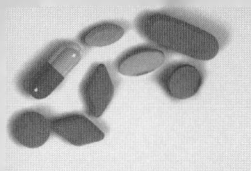

Night-night cancer

A Danish group of forty women have received compensation from their government in recognition that their night-shift work was the probable cause of their cancer.

It is thought that the under-production of the night hormone *melatonin* increased the women's *oestrogen* levels and contributed to their *breast cancer* growth.

Sound advice

'The energy from rock music can peak at 150 decibels. MP3 players are capable of producing sound levels from 60 to 120 decibels. Beware of sounds louder than 85 decibels, which are considered potentially hazardous to your hearing.'

Teddi D. Johnson

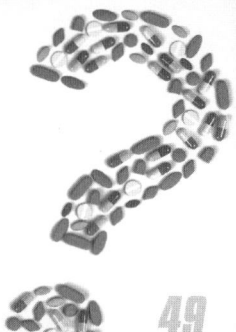

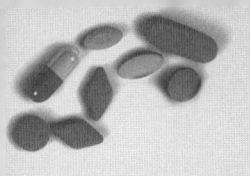

Arterial noise

Evidence in Austria has emerged that steady background traffic noises increase blood pressure, heart rates and stress hormone levels even at non-auditory noise levels.

DNA and AIDS

'Some people with specific genetic variations progress to *AIDS* at twice the average rate of the studied population.'
David Robson

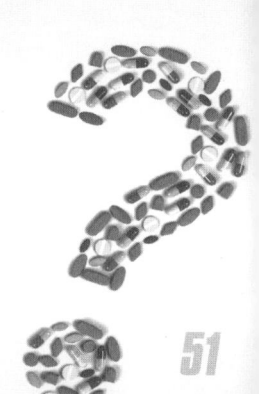

Early diagnosis

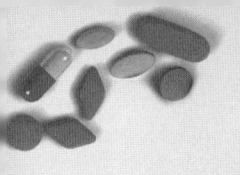

Early diagnosis of infants having *HIV* and treating them early can dramatically reduce death rates, according to a study of 125 *HIV-positive* infants reported in *The New England Journal of Medicine*.

Infants diagnosed early were twice as likely to survive; had a reduced early infant mortality of 76%; with 16% having disease progression.

Safer sex

HIV/AIDS continues to make inroads:

- 33.2m people have *HIV*.
- 270,000 children died of *AIDS* in 2007.
- 6,800 people are newly infected with *HIV* daily.
- There are 15m *AIDS* orphans worldwide.

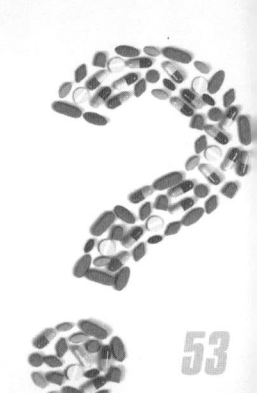

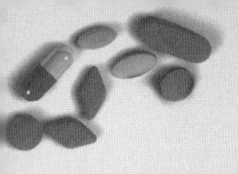

Circumscribed advice

Circumcision protects men from:
- *HIV* (slashing the risk by 50-60%);
- *herpes simplex virus* (reduced by 25%);
- *human papilloma virus* infections (which cause *genital warts*, reducing by 35%).

Microbicidal treatment

A University of Minnesota experiment with the primate version of *HIV (SIV)* may offer hope of blocking *HIV* in humans. The microbicidal – *glycerol monolaurate* – is currently used in food and cosmetics as an *anti-inflammatory*, and was used as a vaginal gel stopping monkeys from being infected with *SIV*. It may also protect against other *STDs*.

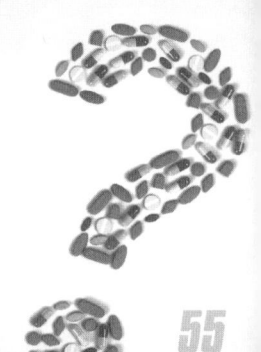

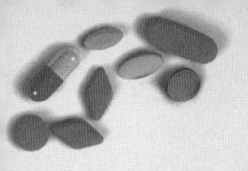

Hoping for a cure

'The miserable have no other medicine
But only hope.'
William Shakespeare

Inherited anxiety

Anxious mums-to-be were 60% more likely to have babies who were also anxious, a study of 6,000 women in Bristol found.

The mothers of 16% of *asthmatic* children had high anxiety during their pregnancy.

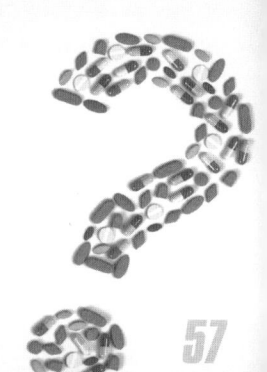

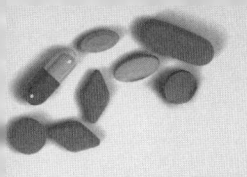

Fighting the blues

'Depression is not an illness – it is a defence which we can use to hold ourselves together when we feel ourselves falling apart.'

Dr Dorothy Rowe

A knock-on effect

'The relation that exists between the mind and the body is very intimate. When one is affected, the other sympathizes. The condition of the mind affects the health to a far greater degree than many realize. Many of the diseases from which men suffer are the result of mental depression. Grief, anxiety, discontent, remorse, guilt, distrust, all tend to break down the life forces and to invite decay and death.'

Ellen White

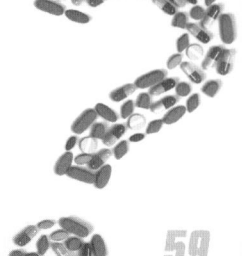

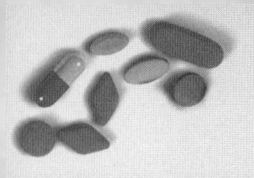

Danger!

'The bow too tensely strung is easily broken.'
Publius Syrus

'Anxiety is the rust of life, destroying its brightness and weakening its power. A childlike and abiding trust in Providence is its best preventive and remedy.'
Tryon Edwards

Lifting the spirit

'Nothing tends more to promote health of body and soul than does a spirit of gratitude and praise. It is a positive duty to resist melancholy, discontented thoughts and feelings – as much a duty as it is to pray.'
Ellen White

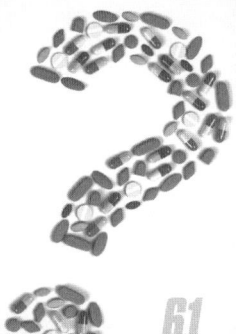

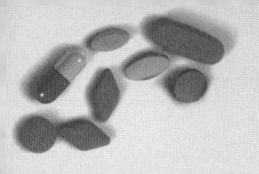

Good grief

'Life is a malady whose one medicine is death.'
Abu'l-'Ala Al-Ma'rri (973-1058)
'Grief is itself a medicine.'
William Cowper (1731-1800)

Premature deaths

- Circa 1 million suicides worldwide every year.
- One suicide every 40 seconds.
- Twenty failed suicide attempts for every successful one.
- Sixty percent increase in suicides worldwide since 1965.

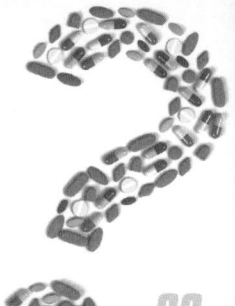

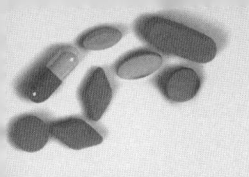

Suicide rates

There has been an unexpected rise in US youth suicides – 18% between 2003 and 2004 and still rising.

'Attention must now be directed toward understanding whether this increase in the youth suicide rate after a decade long decline reflects an emerging public health crisis.'

JAMA

Light living

A study of the *Body Mass Index* of 900,000 adults showed that a *BMI* of 30-35 (moderate obesity) takes two to four years off life expectancy.
Severe obesity claims eight to ten years of life.

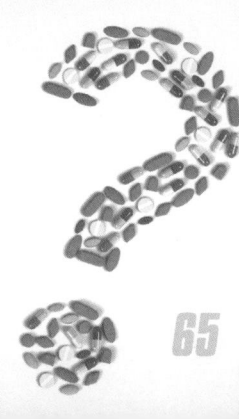

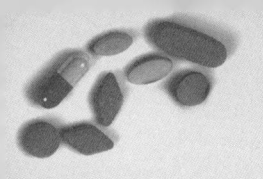

Slim rats

Rats eating ⅓ fewer calories live, on average, 30% longer than force-fed cage-mates.

The excessive eating of the latter increases the production of a protein *(IGF-1)* circulating in the blood and known to cause tumours.

The dangers of inertia

'Lack of activity destroys the good condition of every human being, while movement and methodical physical exercise save it and preserve it.'

Plato

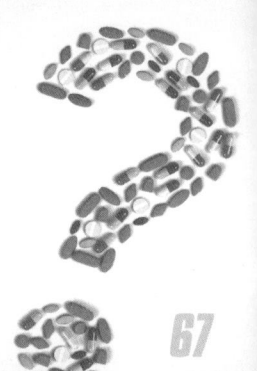

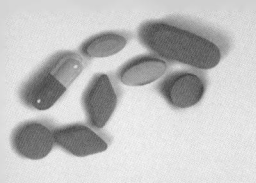

Teletubbies!

'If it weren't for the fact that the TV set and the refrigerator are so far apart, some of us wouldn't get any exercise at all.'
Joey Adams

Trouble ahead!

'Those who think they have no time
for bodily exercise will sooner or later
have to find time for illness.'
Edward Stanley

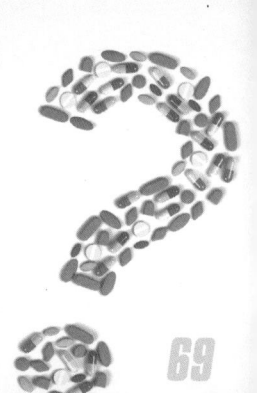

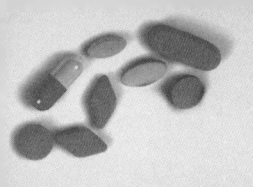

Step it up!

A US study showed the need for men to walk at between 92 and 102 steps a minute and women to walk at 91 to 115 steps a minute to achieve a moderately intense heart workout.

Knocked into shape

Muscle dysmorphia is the name coined for gym fanatics who continue to work out excessively after they have obtained the desired contours.

Ten percent of men and 84% of women suffer the problem of not recognising the finished product.

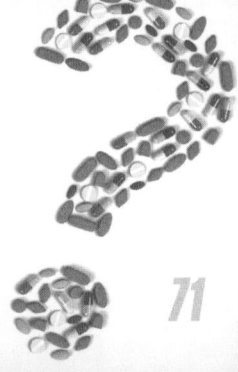

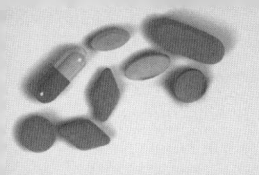

Boneyard

'It's vital people of all ages take regular weight-bearing exercise and eat a balanced, calcium-rich diet, to store "bone in the bank" for their futures.'

National Osteoporosis Society

Run down

Gymnasts and athletes need an optimal exercise
and nutritional regime. Extreme training is out.
Over-exercising can leach vital minerals
and lose vitamin reserves.

This is a particular problem for women athletes
who often stop menstruating early and
suffer *osteoporosis* at a later age.

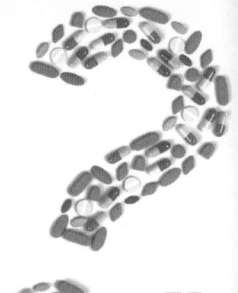

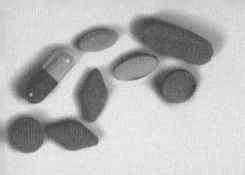

Legging it

Sprinters need perfect legs, so longer legs help. About 50% of our leg muscle fibres twitch for ordinary use, but a runner needs about 80% of his/her fibres for a dash. Runners also need about 50% more oxygen than the average person.

The bear facts

'A bear, however hard he tries,
grows tubby without exercise.'
Winnie the Pooh

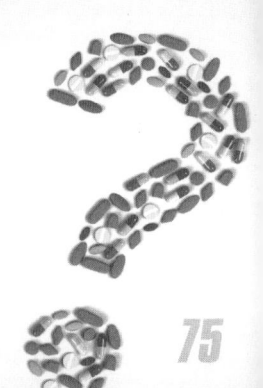

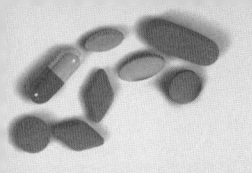

Can't find the time?

'Exercise: you don't have time not to.'
Author unknown

Bearing fruit

'Inactivity is a fruitful cause of disease. Exercise quickens and equalizes the circulation of the blood, but in idleness the blood does not circulate freely, and the changes in it, so necessary to life and health, do not take place. The skin, too, becomes inactive. Impurities are not expelled as they would be if the circulation had been quickened by vigorous exercise, the skin kept in a healthy condition, and the lungs fed with plenty of pure, fresh air.'

Ellen White

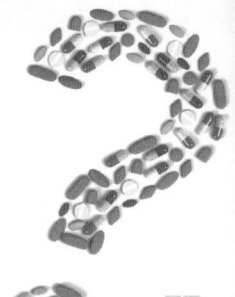

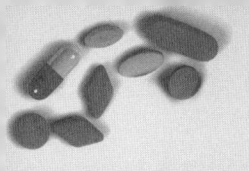

There's love handles...

French researchers have studied body size in 120,000 men and women and concluded that there is a strong link between a large waist measurement and decreased *lung function*.

Fatty tissue may increase inflammatory processes leading to respiratory problems.

... and love Handels

George Frideric Handel was not only big in the music world, but big in any world! He 'paid more attention to his food than is becoming in any man' and was reportedly 'corpulent and unwieldy in his motions'. Handel binged on food and wine to the laughing contempt of his companions.

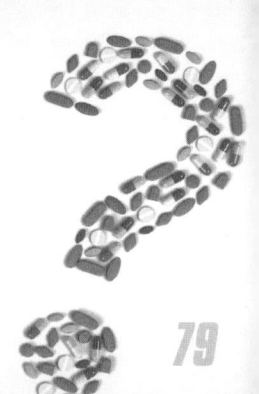

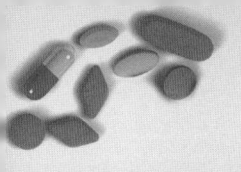

Fatwatch

A wristwatch developed in Japan gives not only the time but a body fat/weight ratio by sending a current to measure the impedance of flesh and then a digital readout on the data feedback.

Chair disease

Sitting in a chair at the office or at home is one of the leading causes of back pain in Americans younger than 45. It is estimated that 8 out of 10 persons will suffer back pain at some point in their lives.

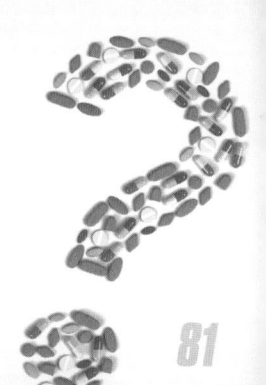

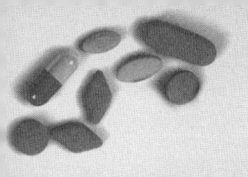

'Terminal' illness . . .

The increasing use of *visual display units* in the workplace and at home has contributed to a range of bodily disorders: muscular problems, headaches, eye strain, inflamed tendons and occasionally skin rashes and disturbed body rhythms.

... and its care

- Take frequent visual breaks and vary the routine.
- Use static exercises (tightening and loosening muscles).
- Deep breathing.
- A regular exercise programme.

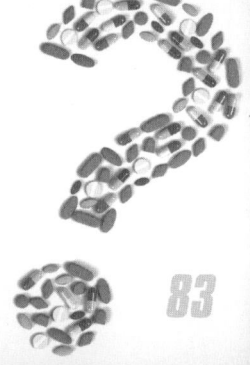

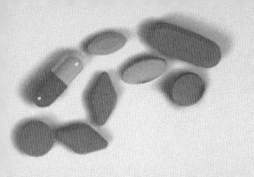

Warm fuzzies

'... if we more often nurtured our companions
and promoted their well-being,
we would suffer less.'

Beatrice Bruteau

Social support

'... social support has been consistently linked, through research, with a low risk of numerous physical and psychiatric illnesses, and with favourable prognosis in sick patients. The absence of social support, on the other hand, is associated with poor health and poor prognosis.'

Richard Totman

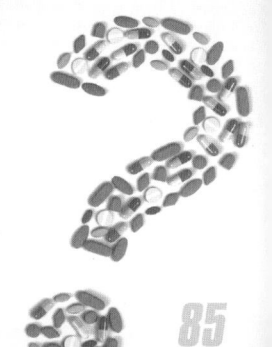

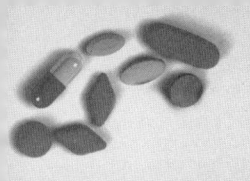

Strength in numbers

'Two people are better than one, because they get more done by working together. If one falls down, the other can help him up. But it is bad for the person who is alone and falls, because no one is there to help.'

Ecclesiastes 4:9, 10, NCV

The value of encouragement

'Treat people as if they were what they ought to be and you help them to become what they are capable of being.'

Goethe

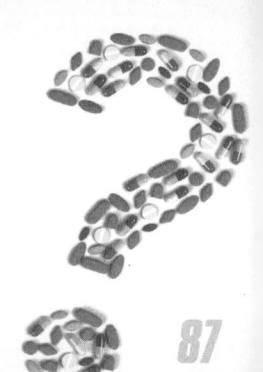

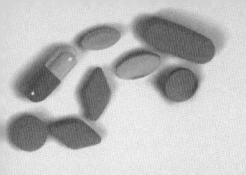

The value of friendship

'Thus nature has no love for solitude,
and always leans, as it were, on some support;
and the sweetest support is found in the
most intimate friendship.'

Cicero

All-round support

With good support: first-time mothers have fewer complications; *renal dialysis* patients rehabilitate more easily; *depression* is reduced; the bereaved have fewer health problems; and the elderly have elevated levels of protective hormones.

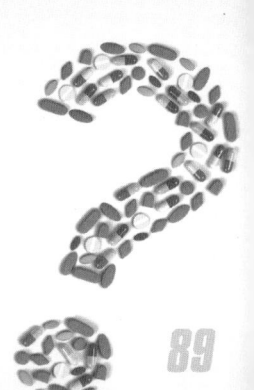

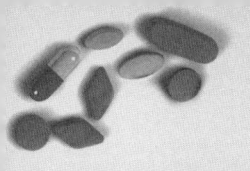

Family conflict

Some research in London showed that family conflict can stint the growth of young children.

Children affected by domestic conflicts are more than twice as likely to be below average height. The stress appears to reduce growth hormone.

Teen killers

'Shootings appear more likely in schools characterised by a high degree of social stratification and low bonding and attachment between teachers and students.'

Traci Wike

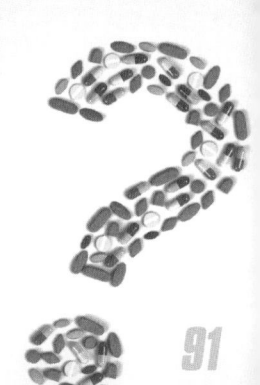

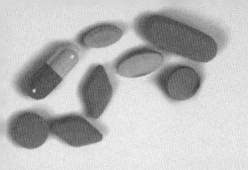

College rage

A study at three US urban colleges showed increased violence rates between partners, friends and acquaintances:

½ experienced relationship violence at some point in their lives

⅓ had experienced violence prior to college

¼ experienced violence while at college

Road rage

Research at De Montfort University showed that stressed drivers are five times more likely to have a fatal accident.

Although other stressors are influencing factors, *road rage* caused drivers to overreact and adopt high-risk behaviours with fatal results.

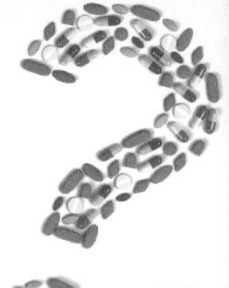

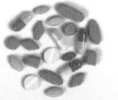

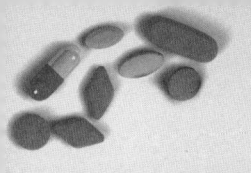

Diabetic siesta

Studies with 16,480 who enjoy a post-prandial nap concluded that 26% of the nappers were at increased risk of developing *Type 2 diabetes*. It is thought the napping somehow interrupted the hormones and mechanisms regulating *insulin* action.

Viral diabetes

Sixty percent of children with *Type 1 diabetes* were found to have *enteroviruses* in their *pancreatic* tissue.

Forty percent of adults with *Type 2 diabetes* also showed signs of the virus in their *insulin-producing* cells.

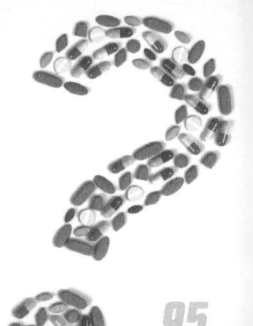

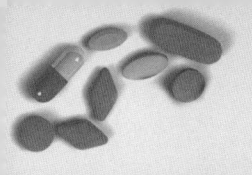

Airborne mercury

Coal-fired power plants in the US emitted 20 tons of *mercury* into the air due to lax federal oversight of the problem. The coal-fired plants are still the largest sources of *mercury* air pollution.

MR SOW MRSA

Studies in Denmark have confirmed that pigs can both carry the *MRSA* and pass it on to humans.

Thirteen of 21 farm workers having *MRSA* reported exposure to pigs. Studies elsewhere suggest that animal-to-human transmission is a reality.

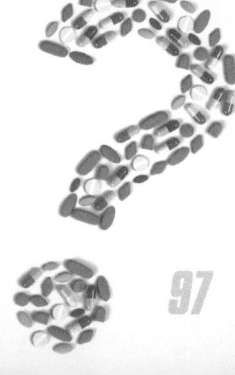

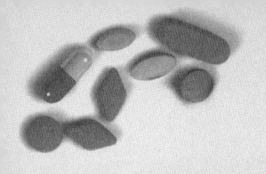

Blind spot

A north London survey showed that 90% of people with *cataracts* were not in touch with eye services.

Over a third of the over 65s had eye problems correctible by glasses or surgery. It is estimated there could be a 20% rise in *partial-sightedness* and *blindness* over the next two decades.

Breaking even!

Annually in the UK there are around 60,000 hip fractures, 50,000 wrist fractures and at least 40,000 vertebral fractures.

A healthy diet using cereals, vegetables, fortified flours and some milk and milk products will go a long way towards reducing these figures.

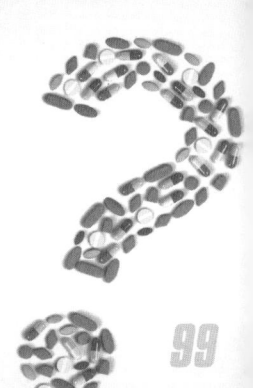

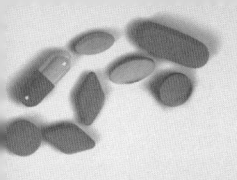

Close companions

In spite of environmental changes and improved personal hygiene worldwide, the head louse *(pediculus capitus)*, body louse *(pediculus humanus corporis)* and the crab louse *(phthirus pubis)* still remain man's closest companions all through history.

Smells good

The human nose has an average smell vocabulary of around 1,000 odours. It is more than capable of picking up the 2,000+ molecules that make up a rose and that change with time of day and the season, and that's just one lovely smell!

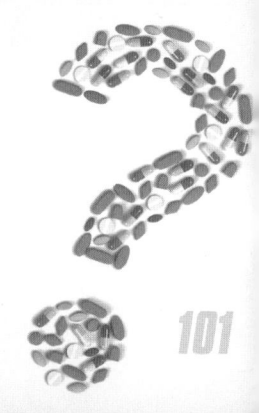

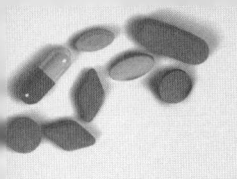

Flight screw!

A University of Bristol study has shown that the brains of aircrew flying through time zones on a regular basis suffer damage.

The women in the study took an average of two weeks to get over jetlag, and they experienced disorientation, exhaustion and sleeplessness.

Poetic allergies

'What linguistic genius set up the sneeze and wheeze

To rhyme so very perfectly with the word for allergies?'

Charlie N. Abbers

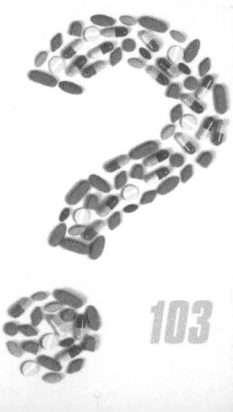

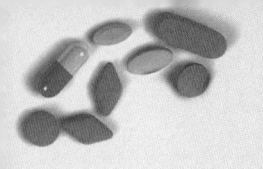

Ruffled fur!

An American company plans to genetically modify cats so that the protein *(Fel d 1)* that causes *allergy* is eliminated.

Mum's lunch

A Danish study of breast milk tastes after giving the women capsules containing compounds common to caraway seed, menthol, banana and liquorice showed that these flavours lasted in the milk for varying lengths of time but could also influence a child's food preferences later on in life.

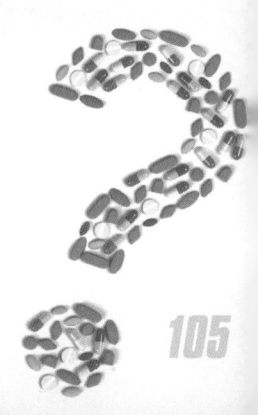

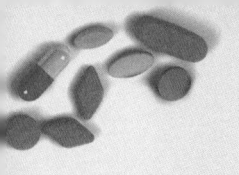

Autistic bowels?

A gene *MET* linked to *autism* also plays a role in repairing damaged gut tissue. In a study of 118 families in which at least one child was *autistic*, a variant of the gene was found, thus confirming a link between *autism* and the unusually high risk of bowel disease suffered by the *autistic*.

Going for broke

Forty-five thousand Swedish men, in a study of lifestyle factors, highlighted the effects of obesity and smoking. The *British Medical Journal* paper stated that being obese at 18 is as dangerous as smoking (each doubles the risk of early death). The obese 18 year olds are five times more likely to die earlier than non-affected peers.

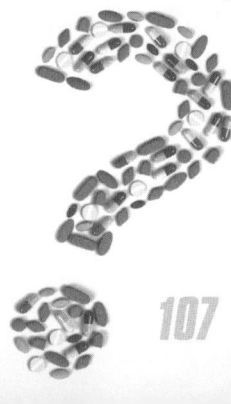

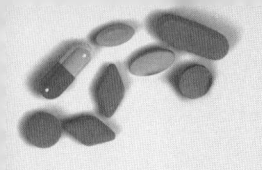

Fast strokes

A link has been established between the incidence of *strokes* and the number of fast-food outlets in a given area.

There were 13% more *strokes* in areas with an average of 33 such eateries.

Grey news

Grey hair, thought to be an effect of ageing, is now believed to be a massive build-up of *hydrogen peroxide*, a by-product of hair wear-and-tear blocking hair's natural pigments.

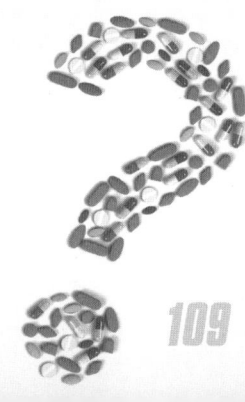

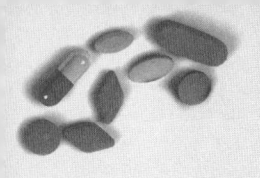

Feeding crime

'There now seems to be sufficient evidence to justify serious attention being given to a serious relationship between food, nutrition and truancy, expulsion from school and antisocial or violent behaviour which may result in criminality.'

Dr J. W. T. Dickerson

Quick fix

Twenty-two popular sports drinks were analysed and found to have high sugar content and the addition of *caffeine*. One of the drinks had 13 level teaspoons of sugar per 300ml bottle. *Caffeine* was often not listed as such but is a naturally occurring ingredient of the *gaurana* commonly used in sports drinks.

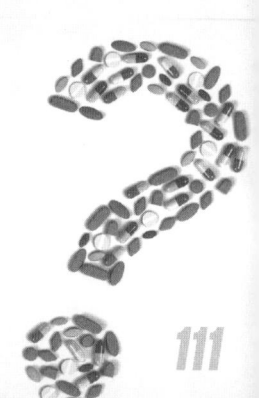

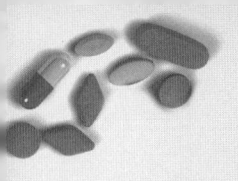

Liver problems

Caffeine raises the level of an enzyme which is used to assess liver function by up to 80% above baseline values, an effect continuing with a 45% increase still present six months later.

Cholesterol and *triglyceride* levels were also raised for an extended period.

Fat substitute

Some manufacturers are using salt to make up for missing fat in lower-fat products. Consequently, salt has been turning up in processed foods where it is least expected – cereal products, cottage cheese, liquorice sticks and bagels.

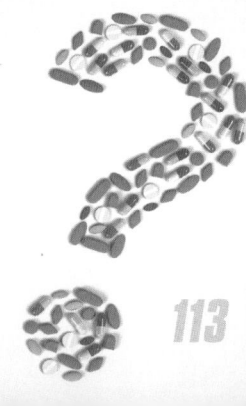

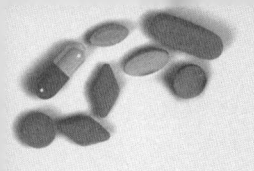

Heart-healthy foods

A new Canadian study confirms that the diet that best protects the heart is vegetables, nuts and the Mediterranean diet, while starchy carbs like white bread and the *trans fats* found in biscuits and French fries is out.

Omega-3s

While fish oils are rich in these *fatty acids*, other sources are nearer to hand.

Nuts and seeds are a good source of *omega-3*, as are green-leaf vegetables such as cabbage and spinach.

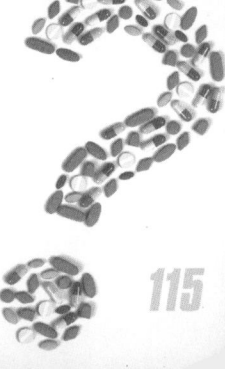

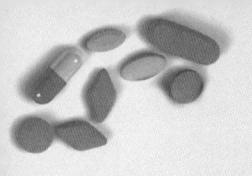

Slow food

Fed up with the commercial clout of fast-food outlets and their adverse effect on health, an Italian journalist – Carlo Petrini – set up the organisation Slow Food in 1989.

It aims to promote traditional ways of farming and cooking, and taking life at a leisurely pace.

Full plates

People who overfill their plates may have more than they bargained for: indigestion, constipation, and a growing weight problem.

Rather than eat less and exercise more, they opt instead for medical treatment at a cost to the NHS of £500 million annually.

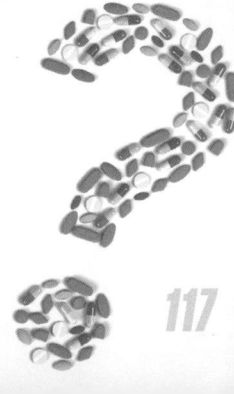

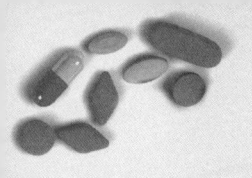

Nuts not to!

'. . . the addition of walnuts to a diet that was already a standard cholesterol-lowering diet, lowered the *blood LDL* [the harmful *cholesterol*] by a further 10% and the mean *blood cholesterol* by 12.4%.'

Professors J. Sabat and G. Fraser

More nuts!

Dr Hu and colleagues studied nut intakes on *coronary heart disease* risk rates in 86,016 UK nurses. After adjusting for specific *CHD* risk factors it was reported that the women had a 35% lower risk if they consumed five units of nuts a week.

(A unit = 1 to 2 ounce intake of any nuts.)

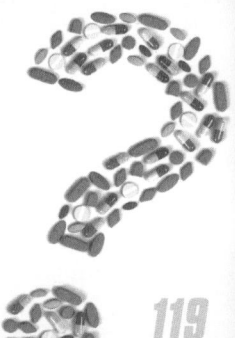

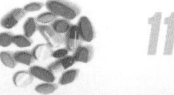

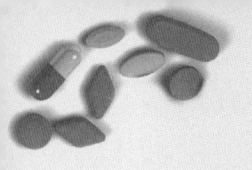

The zinc link

Although it is rare to find *zinc* deficiency, a balance is necessary as it is essential to the chemistry of at least 50 enzymes.

Too little increases a range of illnesses from the common cold to *dwarfism* and *underdeveloped testes*.

Too much can increase *cancer* risk.

Cereal ignorance

The European Cancer Prevention Organisation is trying to encourage a diet rich in high fibre cereals. Cereal's role in cancer protection is not widely known in Europe.

Only 50% of the population are aware of its cancer-risk-reducing potential, the remaining 95% associate it with relieving constipation.

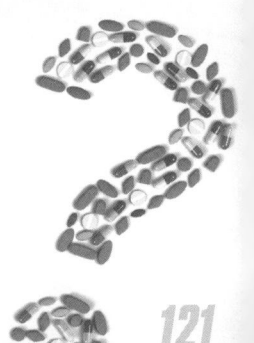

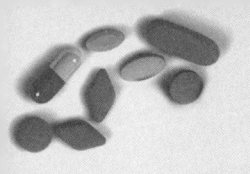

Food for EU

An EU food directive has set limits for the sugar content of processed cereal-based foods for babies and young children.

Biscuits, for example, must not have more than 1.8 grams of added sugar per every 100 kilojoules of energy.

Big misteak!

A committee on the Medical Aspects of Food Policy has shown that 90g of red meat a day increases the risk of *colon* and *breast cancer*. A Department of Health recommendation discourages the use of even this average portion.

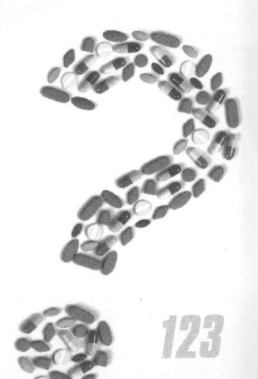

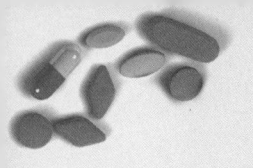

Abracadabra!

'Formerly, when religion was strong and science weak, men mistook magic for medicine; now, when science is strong and religion weak, men mistake medicine for magic.'

Thomas Stephen Szasz

Heaven's highway

'Neurology makes it clear: There's no other way for God to get into your head except through the brain's neural pathways.'
Drs Andrew Newberg and Eugene D'Aquili

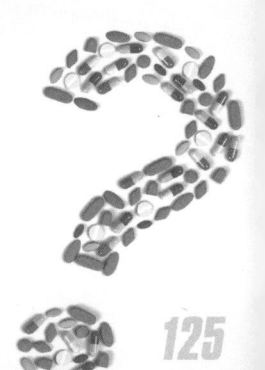

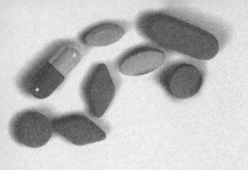

Building damage

'By taking too much food, we not only improvidently waste the blessings of God, provided for the necessities of nature, but do great injury to the whole system. We defile the temple of God; it is weakened and crippled; and nature cannot do its work wisely and well, as God has made provision that it should.'

Ellen White

A second blessing

'Look to your health;
and if you have it, praise God, and value
it next to a good conscience;
for health is the second blessing that
we mortals are capable of;
a blessing that money cannot buy.'

Izaak Walton (1593-1683)

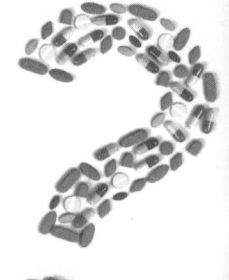

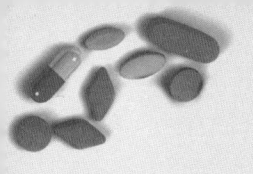

A sacred duty

'It is a duty to know how to preserve the body in the very best condition of health, and it is a sacred duty to live up to the light which God has graciously given.'

Ellen White